HOW TO TRAIN FOR AGING

The Ultimate Endurance Sport

KEVIN THOMAS MORGAN

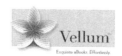

Vellum

Exquisite eBooks. Effortlessly.

How to
Train for Aging

Cover image: *The author completing the Lake Placid Iron-man, at age 68, as the only person to undertake such a race with an abdominal aortic aneurysm stent graft. Nearly 10 years later, now with peripheral vascular disease, he's still training for Iron-man, his beloved sport. Endurance training taught him how to fight the ravages of aging, by adapting to change.*

ALSO BY KEVIN THOMAS MORGAN

The True Story of Plantar Fasciitis

Plantar Fasciitis Has The Wrong Name:

Find Peace of Mind in the Pool

Pain, Good Friend, Bad Master

Autobiography of a Happy Scientist

A Tiny House Fixed My Retirement Cash Flow

Aortic Disease From The Patient's Perspective

Surgery Recovery Guide

Body Meditation for Optimal Movement

Changing the Way You Move

DEDICATION

I dedicate this book to four remarkable athletes.

Nigel, *my youngest son, and experienced Ironman Triathlete, who inspired me to try this fascinating sport.*

Frits with an "s," *who is sorely missed. Thanks for the "Ironman Training Secret Sauce," my friend.*

Rory, *who taught me how to suffer on the bike.*

Bob Scott, *who beat me three times in the Eagleman Half Ironman race, while in his early 80s with heart stents, a gentleman and truly inspiring master of Aging.*

EPIGRAPH

Aging is not lost youth but a new stage of opportunity and strength.

– Betty Friedan

FOREWORD

There is a huge body of knowledge supporting the belief that age changes are characterized by increasing Entropy ...

– Leonard Hayflick

Selected links to the *FitOldDog video channel* referred to in the text are provided at *prepareforaging.com*.

MY DAY

I wake up in my tiny house around 4:00 a.m. and put on the kettle for a cup of tea. Two cups of tea, in fact. I love this time of day. The stars fade as the chatter of insects dissolves into the dawn chorus.

I feed my ginger cat, Cat, and yellow lab, Willbe, and read for a while. Once it's light, I check what needs doing in the vegetable garden, and collect some food for breakfast. After a tasty homegrown meal, I start my daily writing tasks. Mid-morning, Willbe and I take a walk to a coffee shop. Willbe gets a treat and I enjoy my daily cup of coffee, as I chat with the locals or read a book on my phone.

I do love to read, both fiction and non-fiction.

Sometime during the day, I'll undertake one or two planned workouts. These often include a run with Willbe. If so, I head for the local running track. No need to change, as I live in running gear. It's an old habit that still works in my mid-70s. Wicking shirt, running shorts, light zero-rise shoes.

At the track, I adjust the settings of my sports watch to record distance, pace and heart rate. Then off we go for a run of several miles. Four laps of the track make a mile. Why the track, which many find boring? Because there's a smooth running surface and few interruptions.

We run 100 yards, 200 yards, 250 and then we stop.

I stand immobile on my left leg, as pain surges through my right calf. Willbe sits patiently at my side. He knows the drill. I glance at my watch as it calculates average running pace. It grows from 9 minutes and 30 seconds per mile, through 10 minutes, 11 minutes and finally 18 minutes and 20 seconds per mile. This is not much better than a brisk walking pace.

Time was moving, but we were not.

As we wait that calf gradually relaxes, the pain subsides, and we run another 250 or 300 yards. Again, I'm forced to stop and repeat the calf pain procedure. This allows life-giving blood to flow through a partially blocked artery in my right leg, into oxygen-starved calf muscles.

As the mileage increases our mile time improves to 14 minutes and 12 seconds per mile. I'm getting closer to my goal of 13 minutes and 40 seconds per mile. If I can average 13 minutes and 40 seconds per mile for 26.2 miles, I will achieve a 6-hour marathon time. Then I'll be ready to sign up for another Ironman race, which starts with a 2.4-mile swim, then a 112-mile bike ride, finishing with a full 26.2-mile marathon. Yep! It's a long day, but I love it.

You have to complete such races in less than 17 hours. If I can run the marathon in six hours, I should be able to finish an Ironman race in under 15 hours. This would give me a chance to qualify for the World Ironman Championships in Kona, Hawaii, where I hope to take my friend Frits's ashes along. Frits always wanted to qualify for Kona, before his untimely death two years ago.

If I can qualify, and there's no guarantee, Frits will get to do the race in spirit. When I suggested this idea to his widow, Machteld, she said with a tear that she loved the idea, as a way of keeping Frits's memory alive.

Furthermore, it won't be all about me, and I like that.

To think that in 2009, I qualified for the Boston Marathon, in Charlotte, North Carolina, with a time of four hours and seven minutes, with an average pace of 9 minutes and 27 seconds per mile. Now I'm struggling to reach a 13:40 pace. But I'm a decade older, and a man has to know his limitations.

But that's no damned reason not to try.

My ongoing training will slowly encourage the growth of new blood vessels around that partially blocked popliteal artery in my right leg. This blockage is due to hardening of my arteries, or arteriosclerosis, which is related to my genetically high blood fat levels. The muscle conditioning from my ongoing training, combined with modifying the way I run to spare those calf muscles as best I can, will also contribute to my progress.

Oddly enough, peripheral arterial disease in my legs has no impact on cycling or swimming performance.

Ironman triathlon training in my 50s, which was no easy task, dramatically improved my genetically unhealthy blood fat profile. This endurance sport also saved my life from an abdominal aortic aneurysm, in my mid-60s. Even this *life-threatening aneurysm (link available at prepareforaging.com)* didn't stop my Ironman training. I did have to modify the way I moved to protect the stent graft that now holds my aorta together. When it comes to running, the aortic aneurysm, though more danger-ous, turned out to be less challenging than peripheral arterial disease in my legs.

Go figure!

Fortunately, all my life I'd been training my body and my mind for the health challenges of Aging. I just didn't know it. A lifetime of mental and physical activity is now enabling me to adapt to yet another challenge, this being the secret of survival.

I have no complaints. I'm 76 years old and still train-ing. And I've had a great life so far. I'm very blessed, and what's a little pain if I can return to my favorite sport.

BACK TO THE TRACK.

Once the run is completed, I go through a stretching routine. If you don't stretch after a run your muscles become really tight, increasing risk of injuries. Later that day I'll do a swim in the pool, some weight training at the gym, or a bike ride on the roads. It depends on my training plan.

Then back to reading, writing, and general life chores.

REMEMBER THESE WISE WORDS AS YOU AGE:

It is not the strongest of the species that survives, nor the most intelligent. It is the one that is most adaptable to change.

– Charles Darwin

It's been a good day so far, because once again I've fought back against the ravages of Entropy.

But I didn't do this on my own.

I had the help and support and training of many people, from family and friends to coaches, training partners, and body-movement specialists, and, "Yes!" remarkable doctors and surgeons who repair my Aging body, to keep it on the Ironman course, though they do express their reservations about that!

You just don't do it on your own, any more than a single soldier can win a battle.

WHAT YOU NEED TO KNOW

When it comes to Aging, it's important to realize that there are two forces at work, one negative and the other positive. The negative or destructive force is called *Entropy*. The counter force, used by life, is *Syntropy*. They are in conflict, and you can influence the outcome of this conflict by training for Aging.

This book is about how to train to fight Entropy, as it attempts to ruin your old age. You do this by making an effort to engage actively in life, physically, mentally, emotionally and spiritually, as the years go by.

My goal is for you to tell Entropy to piss off, while encouraging Syntropy into your life.

WHAT DO I KNOW?

This book is about training for the ultimate endurance sport, Aging, based on my diverse range of sporting activities, including Ironman triathlons, and as an enthusiast of body-awareness and body movement training.

But what do I know?

Endurance Sports: I spent the last quarter century training for the race known as Ironman. It's 140.6 miles of swimming, biking and running, all in one day, all under your own steam. This was preceded by a life-time of other sporting endeavors, including water-polo, racquetball, skiing, weight lifting and martial arts, under excellent instructors. I ran the Boston Marathon in 2009, no mean feat for someone lacking a runner's body type. I enjoyed them all, and I'm still training. I'm a damned lucky old guy.

Aging: I first encountered this response to the ministrations of Entropy in my early forties. Aging had begun it's relentless attacks. *I couldn't read a damned thing without my glasses.* Then came my abdominal aortic aneurysm in my 60s, with ballooning of the biggest artery in my body. If it burst, which it was ready to do, I'd be dead in minutes or less. I dodged that bullet due to my pathology and body-awareness training.

More recently, in my 70s, I've developed peripheral arterial disease, which impairs blood flow to my lower legs, especially my feet when I run. Have I given up Ironman because of this? No way! I'm finding a way to work around the problem.

I'm engaging all the Syntropy I can get.

Like any older person, I'm stiffer in the morning when I get up, I have to avoid injuries at all costs, it takes me longer to build strength and speed, and longer to recover from workouts. In spite of all my training, I tend to feel old some days. That is when I allow my enemy, Entropy, to get a look in, which is rare, but becoming tougher for me to resist. That resistance is the subject of this book.

Aging as an Endurance Sport: I know that training is essential for endurance sports. I know that Aging is the ultimate endurance sport. I know that Aging is the result of Entropy.

Fighting Entropy: It is clear that appropriate training is essential for enduring Aging successfully. You have to make an effort. You have to play your part. You can't afford to remain passive as Entropy mounts its offensive on your life and the joy of living.

Gird your loins for battle.

LIFE IS FOR LIVING

Does it take the harsh light of disaster to show a person's true nature?

> — Jean-Dominique Bauby, who went bravely through a living hell at the end of his life.

When I reached my 50th. birthday, I became a little depressed. I felt as though I was staring old age in the face.

What was my problem?

I was being tricked by Entropy.

In 2010, at age 67, with my newly diagnosed abdominal aortic aneurysm, I felt as though I'd gone from

Ironman triathlete scientist to aortic cripple. Essentially overnight!

Since both those events, my 50th. birthday and that blasted aneurysm, I successfully changed the nature of my scientific career several times. Now I'm learning how to make a living as a writer, a real endurance sport, but not as tough as Aging.

I still see adventures in my future. New battles to fight, mountains to climb, things to see and learn. I don't want to die leaving any stone unturned.

That said, I tend to live in today, rather than dwelling on memories of the past or dreaming of the future.

I wake up each morning and think, *What's it to be today?*

Have you ever ridden through Paris, France, in the morning rush hour traffic, on the back of a motorbike, going up to 70 miles per hour, dodging between cars and pedestrians, around the *Arc de Triomphe* and other famous sites, on your way from the outskirts of the city to the Gare du Nord, for the train to London. I did the other day. How did that come about?

I asked if I could.

My friend Claire's nice boyfriend, Nicolas, said, *bien entendu* (sure), and went in search of a crash helmet that would fit on my rather large bullet of a head.

I could have said to myself, *I'm too old for such fool-ishness.*

I'm pleased to say that I ignored Entropy's whisperings in my mind, as it tried to talk me out of this exciting adventure.

Come to think of it, if you haven't done so already, learning another language and its culture is a great adventure. It's never too late to try. You may not become fluent, but you will receive the appreciation of the people who speak that language. They are glad to see you try. To see you show an interest in them.

That's what humans like and maybe need. Others to show an interest in their lives.

Don't be enticed away from such excitement, toward your grave, by the siren's voice of Entropy.

Take some chances.

A life without risk is no life at all.

JEAN DOMINQUE BAUBY WAS RIGHT.

For me, personally, it turned out that my aortic aneurysm was a life changer, it changed for the better. It got me more in touch with my feelings, friends and family, less interested in social and financial success, it gave me a mission in life, to help others in the same situation. As my hero, Jean Dominique Bauby, suggested, that, "It does take the harsh light of disaster to show a person's true nature."

My life changed for the better, changed for the better by what one might interpret as a disaster, a major health challenge.

Sorry, Entropy, you failed to take me down.

SECTION ONE - KNOW THINE ENEMY

If you know the enemy and know yourself, you need not fear the result of a hundred battles. If you know yourself but not the enemy, for every victory gained you will also suffer a defeat. If you know neither the enemy nor yourself, you will succumb in every battle.

– Sun Tzu, The Art of War

Entropy

Defining your Enemy

WHAT ENTROPY DOES

- Entropy can blind your awareness of yourself as you age.
- Entropy will distract you from working on your flexibility.
- Entropy loves it when you have poor posture.
- Entropy has no interest in your core training.
- Entropy will try to stop you learning new things as you age.
- Entropy doesn't want you to find and fix your misalignments.
- Entropy will fight against your physical and mental conditioning.
- Entropy has no interest in your emotions.
- Entropy will resist your attempts to think clearly.
- Entropy doesn't want you to master healthy drinking.

- Entropy loves it when you eat crap food.
- Entropy is delighted when you fail to taper before an event.
- Entropy has no interest in your transition skills.
- Entropy is no coach, and doesn't want you to find one.
- Entropy won't reward you, except with death.
- Entropy will unbalance your center.
- Entropy will fight tooth and nail against training for Aging, the true endurance sport.

But you are life, and life turns Entropy on its head.

THE ENEMY

Entropy

A thermodynamic quantity representing the unavailability of a system's thermal energy for conversion into mechanical work, often interpreted as the degree of disorder or randomness in the system (*Author's interpretation - Everything in the universe is turning into background heat radiation, aka Heat Death*).

The second law of thermodynamics says that Entropy always increases with time. (*Author's interpretation - We're screwed, gradually disintegrating, like a rusty old car.*)

Hell! I've had some great times in rusty old cars. Trips into the countryside, picnics in rest-stops, remarkable meals cooked out of the back.

It would appear that most physicists today agree about Entropy.

Life has other ideas.

ENTROPY AND EXCITEMENT

Entropy wants to kill your excitement. What could be more alive than excitement. Remember when you fell in love, or made a great pass in football, or got an A in a quiz, or that attractive person said, "Yes," when you asked them out. That's excitement! Entropy wants to take that away from you. I don't care how old you are, you are not too old to feel excitement.

Entropy wants to steal that away.

Entropy wants to eliminate your excitement for good.

ENTROPY AND ENJOYMENT

Damn, I do enjoy life. You? What do you enjoy? Seeing your kids, a good hand in poker, a beautiful sunset? A real achievement at work? A solid workout completed, a race well-run, maybe even better than last time? Being greeted by your dog as you come home from work, admiring your new, or not so new, car? An evening with friends, some admiring comments from others? Who knows what you enjoy, but you know?

Entropy wants to spoil your enjoyment. Entropy wants to take it all away and make it worth nothing, zero, nada, turn it into background heat radiation.

ENTROPY AND BEING ALIVE

As an older triathlete, running through a thunderstorm in a foot of water, damn, I feel alive. Yes! Alive. The sense of being out there, in nature, in touch with the earth, full of life. Full of living life to the full. It feels ecstatic. Soaking wet, with flashes of lighting all around me, but I'm out there. Often alone, oddly enough. How does one describe it?

It's a feeling of doing sh*t.

Entropy doesn't want you to do exciting sh*t. No siree!

ENTROPY AND DISMAY

When I screwed up my knee again, because I hadn't yet learned how to run safely, I was dismayed. I was in a state of consternation. A state of distress. I was unhappy. Then, I was reminded of a friend who gave me some sage advice, while I was going through a difficult personal challenge. He said, *Kevin, this means you're alive. You can't feel good all the time. If you don't feel bad, how can you feel it's opposite, good, joyful, lively, happy, all those not bad things? Life would be flat, like the weather in California. Appreciate feeling bad. Enjoy it!*

In contrast to my friend, Entropy didn't want me to realize that my state of dismay was a positive experience. Entropy wanted me to dwell on it. Marinade in it. Become angry and resentful. Simmer on a low flame. Blame the world.

Entropy isn't my friend.

ENTROPY AND EXHAUSTION

Have you ever been so exhausted you could cry. You feel like lying down and never getting up. You just can't do it anymore. You want to give up. Poor you! You just want life to be easier. Why isn't life easier? Why does life always beat you down, and *why can't you see a damned thing without your glasses,* it's not fair? Maybe you'll take a break and finish this tomorrow. Have another drink. Chill out. Watch some more TV.

Entropy loves it when you have another glass of wine and a cigarette.

Entropy loves it when you continue to veg out in front of the TV.

Entropy loves it when you feel you can't go on.

"But I feel so tired."

Whatever!

ENTROPY AND AWE

Have you ever felt awe at something, like the beauty of a flower or the stars in the sky? A hummingbird, a fresh tomato straight off the plant and warm in your hand, of a hot summer's eve? Awe is a remarkable feature of being alive. Awe comes with a sense of spirituality and respect, mixed with fear and humility. Awe takes your breath away. Like the person you are in love with.

For instance, try riding a category one hill climb on a bicycle. It feels like riding your bike through a brick wall. Afterwards you will have a sense of awe as you watch the cyclists in the Tour de France scale hills that would make you cry, as if they are nothing. They climb them fast and furious. That's what awe feels like to me.

Sometimes awe requires your personal experience in order for you to appreciate what is going on before your eyes.

I don't feel awe for Entropy.

I feel disdain.

Beaten by sunshine and clever chemistry in little bags of water.

Yes! You are made out of little bags of water, called cells, built of sunshine and Syntropy.

Entropy wants to diminish your sense of awe, to take your awe away.

No way!

Life impresses me, but Entropy is a loser.

ENTROPY AND VICTIMHOOD

Ever feel like the victim, that life isn't treating you right, nothing is going well, and it's not your fault, it's the government's fault, industry's fault, your neighbor, your Mom who did this to you. There is nothing you can do about these people, they have it in for you, and you always did your best, you didn't cause all these problems in your life, THEY did, you hate them, you really do, and it's not your fault, you're the victim of a conspiracy against you.

Entropy loves this stuff, because it traps you in the life of a victim, and it spreads distrust and hate, just what Entropy wants.

ENTROPY AND FEAR

Fear is the big one. See all those older people shuffling around, scared they might fall. Do you want to go there before your time?

If you're scared you won't do stuff. You'll play it safe. You'll not want to lose your life. It's too precious. In fact, your life is so precious you don't want to risk it by actually living. Entropy loves the way you think. But then you would be throwing away all the work that life has been doing for a few billion years. You would be throwing it away out of fear.

When I train in the mountains on my road bike, I feel fear. I feel the fear of crashing on a long bike descent. You should try taking a bunch of hairpin bends on a racing bicycle at 40 to 50 miles an hour. One bad turn and you'd careen off the road and be dead in the trees, literally dead. Scared? Sure! But you don't have time for it, you're too busy obeying the first rule of cycling.

Keep the rubber side down.

This is not the fear Entropy likes. It's the fear of exhilaration, fear laced with excitement and a little terror. It's the fear that comes from being alive, damn it.

A life without risk, and thus some fear, is no life at all. Want to do something exciting, but risky?

Entropy will try to talk you out of it.

F*ck Entropy

ENTROPY AND LAUGHTER

Entropy doesn't want you to laugh.

Remember rolling on the ground, splitting your sides, with laughter? I did that once, while reading a book on a plane. I was doubled up, reading *Portnoy et son Complexe*, by Philip Roth, translated from American English into French, by Henri Robillot. No offense meant, Mr. Roth, but it's definitely better in French. I wasn't embarrassed, I was too busy having incapacitating abdominal spasms. Why do I remember that after almost 40 years? It was so damned funny.

See! Learning another language is a great way to fight Entropy.

This kind of laughter appears less frequently as I age. Maybe I'm getting old. Maybe I think I'm old. Maybe I'm giving into Entropy.

No way!

I can't wait to laugh like that again, to gainsay Entropy.

ENTROPY AND PAIN

Ever wonder if you can continue to face the pain of life anymore. Whether you've had enough. Entropy is waiting with open arms for you to throw in the towel, no need to go another round, no need to suffer, just let it go, who needs pain?

I'll tell you who needs pain.

You do!

Pain is part of living, it is part of doing anything worthwhile. Pain is what we overcome to develop depth of character. To change for the better. People who avoid pain at all cost are giving up their life to Entropy.

It's your call.

Entropy will smile with delight to see you so soon.

ENTROPY NEVER GIVES UP

Entropy wants to kill your enjoyment of all these feelings and the activities that go with them. Entropy is invisible, but it's working to destroy you all the time. The battle against Entropy becomes tougher later in life, as Entropy squeezes you tighter and tighter, trying to crush the joy out of you. But you have experience. You have courage earned from many previous battles.

You are life, and life has been kicking Entropy's ass successfully for eons.

ENTROPY AND RETIREMENT

Entropy would prefer that you did not plan ahead for your later years. Entropy doesn't care if you stay in shape physically, mentally, emotionally, spiritually. "Why bother," says Entropy, you are getting ready for retirement. You'll save and save and save so you can sit around, play golf, just not work any more.

You've been looking forward to retirement, all your working life. Get rid of the job, take it easy for a change. No need for all that exhausting life stuff, driving you along to achieve things, anymore. Why bother, when you can hang out?

Train for Aging? Are you joking? You mean exercise? Challenge my mind? Find a mission in life? I've done my time, so f*ck that.

It's my turn to take a break, I'll be retired at last.

Entropy can't wait for you to retire.

SECTION TWO - KNOW THYSELF

Syntropy

The tendency towards energy concentration, increase in differen-
tiation, complexity and structures. These are the mysterious
properties of life.

– Ulisse Di Corpo and Antonella Vannini,
Introduction to Syntropy

Life

Defining Yourself

WHAT IS LIFE?

Life is wet and dynamic.

> − Howard Berg, *Random walks in biology.*

Life is a fire that burns in a special way.
Life's fire makes stuff.
Life is a dancing fire, a dance of joy.
Life is a fiery song.
Life is a thoughtful fire.
Life is a naysayer of flames.
Life is a warrior, burning with the power of Syntropy.
Life is an athlete, an endurance athlete.
Life has been beating back Entropy for eons.

You are that warrior, life.
You are that athlete, life.

Train to fight your Internal Enemy, Entropy.

Train to fight your External Enemy, Entropy.

Laugh and cry and dance as you do battle, as you compete in your personal game of life, in your fight to the life against Entropy.

WHAT LIFE DOES

Unlike your enemy, Entropy, life creates instead of destroying. Maybe we aren't so screwed as most physicists liked to think, due to Syntropy.

Is this real, this Syntropy stuff? Is the Earth the center of the Universe with the stars being pushed around us by celestial creatures, is the Earth flat, is there such a thing as SpaceTime? Do we understand anything? Or are our ideas only useful metaphors. Who cares, as long as they work and help us to understand where we fit in and how best to live our lives?

Since all this Entropy Thermodynamics stuff was written, along came relativity, which is weird, and then quantum mechanics, even weirder, then Feynman diagrams and time going backwards, followed by chaos and complexity theories, and strange attractors.

The famous physicist, Schrödinger, said that life lives on negative Entropy. No disrespect intended, but to call it negative Entropy, is like calling Love, negative Hate. Fortunately there is a better term, Syntropy.

The time going backwards thing, when it comes to Syntropy, is called *retrocausality,* and it's what permits the creation of life.

Entropy and Syntropy exist in a state of balance, with Entropy working to kill life, and life playing to defy Entropy.

You are life. You kick Entropy in the butt using Syntropy.

Life is a wonderful mystery, of which you are a warrior athlete, who fights Entropy tooth and nail.

Yes, you. So you have training to do, and that training must be fun, to irritate the crap out of Entropy.

SCREW ENTROPY

The challenge of life is: how to increase Syntropy and reduce Entropy by remaining active?

— Ulisse Di Corpo, Antonella Vannini

Entropy wants to destroy your enjoyment of the flavors of wonderful food and wonderful sex, or satisfaction with a job well done, or a calm moment over a cup of tea, or even the anticipation of your next adventure.

Yes! But you are an endurance athlete armed with Syntropy, so you can enjoy Aging, in spite of it all.

You can do it!

YOU ARE DANCE

You are the dance of life, a dance of joy. Life is also a dance of despair, of pain, of fear, of delight. Life is always moving, in all of it's forms, one way or another life is moving. The dance of life is a dangerous dance, but it's the only dance it knows. Life has to beat a formidable enemy. A powerful enemy. An enemy that never sleeps. An enemy that is always watching, ready to devour life itself.

The enemy of life is Entropy, the great destroyer.

So dance the dance of life for all you're worth.

YOU ARE SONG

Life is one grand, sweet song, so start the music.

– Ronald Reagan

There is power in music. Power to make life. Power to take life's burning fire, fire from sunlight, and turn it into the remarkable song of life, the song of the hero. That song is your body, your cells, your friends and family. You don't think you and they are music? Look again, see the beauty of the most remarkable music, the most remarkable piece of Art in the Universe.

You!

Sing the song of your life.

Sing it to Entropy.

Entropy will quake and fail.

YOU ARE GRATEFULNESS

Your body is a huge community. An integrated community. A community of trillions of cells. Each cell has a precious life. Millions of these cells give up their lives for you each day, every minute, every second. You are alive because you are sculpted, yes, sculpted by death. Sculpted by the voluntary death of cells.

Death is your ally in the battle against life-killing Entropy. Look at your hands. Their magical structure, and consider what they do for you. Your fingers only exist because of death. Death of the cells that would have bound your fingers together into a single mass as you grew in your mother's womb. These cells died in order that you could have fingers. When you look at your hands, thank those cells that died for you before you were born.

Entropy hates gratefulness.

Be grateful.

YOU ARE NOT ALONE

Your community of cells, of which you are made, could not survive without your external community. Your family, friends, village, country, continent, the entire Biosphere of all living plants, animals and other creatures, are precious members of your extended family. Many, including myself, consider the living surface of planet Earth, the Biosphere, Gaia, to be conscious, aware. Gaia created you, and now it is time for you to pay back, to do your part for all living creatures on this planet, to do your work of fighting, of racing, against Entropy, by using your old age experience and skills to make things better for all of us.

This will give your old age meaning, a feeling of warmth and contentment, your Syntropic struggles would then have real value. Your struggles will help all other members of life on Planet Earth to feel that they are not alone. So do your part, fight, fight for your life and the life of the planet.

Be a good community member, a foot soldier, an athlete, in the race against Entropy.

YOU ARE THOUGHT

Somehow life arrived, no-one really knows how, and single cells were formed, then they worked together to make complex structures, of which you are one, one composed of many other complex structures, including your brain, which thinks. I suspect that even single cells think, in their single cell ways. I don't think that thinking only occurs in your brain, it occurs throughout your body, throughout the entire living surface of this planet..

Make your thoughts the enemy of Entropy, by thinking positive, creative, never giving up your life's meaning, thoughts.

Let your thoughts be good friends and allies of Syntropy in your battle with Entropy.

YOU ARE THE NAYSAYER.

The naysayer, Entropy, which lives within you and around you, tells you it can't be done. The naysayer tells you everything is pointless because all life dies in the end. You reply that life has been living for several billion years, and life is still dancing, and singing, and feeling and living. The naysayer, the Worm Tongue in your mind, will try to talk you out of dancing and singing and thinking and building and loving. But you are a warrior who can destroy the naysayer, the naysayer in your mind, in your body, in your heart, by fighting Entropy with your mind and your body and your heart.

You are life, you are the hero.

YOU ARE FEELINGS

Feelings are powerful. Feelings provide the energy that powers your ship of life, your body. Combined with reason, your rudder, you can achieve great things in the battle against Entropy. You can promote life, but only if you harness your feelings, and feed the good wolf of your soul. Then the power of your feelings can join the battle against the destroyer, Entropy.

With the help of your friend, ally and companion, Syntropy, you can change the world, even in your later years.

YOU ARE THE TRICKSTER

If your enemy is hungry, feed him; if he is thirsty, give him something to drink. In doing this, you will heap burning coals on his head.

Christian Bible, Proverbs 25:21-22

Life is a trickster, it survives with artifice. You, life, trick Entropy by cheating death, by burning sunlight you dance, build community, think and feel and create good things into old age, in spite of the ravages of Entropy. You overcome Entropy's destruction by living. Living life to the full, with laughter, even in the face of death. You are the laughing, loving, fiery warrior endurance athlete, who keeps the dance going, dancing in sunbeams.

You give the middle finger to Entropy. You shake your fist at Entropy. Then as the trickster, you love Entropy as your friend, because Entropy hates love.

Destroy that hate with your love. Love is a greater power than Entropy. Use love as your weapon against Entropy by loving all living and non-living things.

Have kind feelings towards Entropy as a fellow traveler, and Entropy will hate you for it, because Entropy will know that you cannot be tricked by Entropy's wily ways of destruction.

You are life!

OVERCOMING ENTROPY

Bob Scott had several heart stents in his late 60s, and went on to set age-group records in the World Ironman Championships in Kona, Hawaii, in his 70s.

Rick, my swim training buddy, was told 10 years ago that he would be dead in four years, due to an autoimmune disease. This progressed to include type I diabetes. A few months ago, and not dead, he completed the Austria Ironman in a respectable time.

Benjamin Carry ran the New York City Marathon, with his heart surgeon, who had a tougher time than Benjamin in the run, after open heart surgery for an ascending aortic aneurysm.

With the inspiration of such people, and many others, plus the help of remarkable surgeons, I overcame an abdominal aortic aneurysm in 2010, and went on continue Ironman training. This was followed by peripheral arterial disease in my mid-70s, but I've just signed up for the 2020, Florida Ironman.

How do we do such things?

We train for Aging! We fight Entropy tooth and nail.

The next section will tell you how you can, too.

SECTION THREE - TRAINING FOR AGING

It is one thing to study war and another to live the warrior's life.

— Telamon of Arcadia

Syntropy *versus* Entropy

Defeating Your Enemy

MEDICAL DISCLAIMER

As a veterinarian, I do not provide medical advice to human animals. If you undertake or modify an exercise program, consult your medical advisers before doing so. Undertaking activities pursued by the author does not mean that he endorses your undertaking such activities, which is clearly your decision and responsibility.

Be careful and sensible, please.

Kevin Thomas Morgan aka FitOldDog
Old Dogs in Training, LLC.
Carrboro,
North Carolina,
USA

November, 2019

WHY TRAIN?

As a life form you are a warrior athlete fighting against the destructive force of Entropy.

That means that you cannot sit back and let Syntropy do all the work, when it comes to making Aging meaningful.

No Way!

You have endurance training to do, physical, intellectual, emotional, and spiritual training.

If you want to get started, now, I've provided a simple training plan as Chapter 49, but I recommend reading all of the material before you start. It won't take you long, and the details could be important for your success as an older warrior athlete, fighting the ravages of Entropy with your ally and friend, Syntropy.

Rock on, but finish this book first.

If you really want to see the benefits of training as you age, go to the "Why Train?" tab at prepareforaging.com.

Each Train for Aging section is followed by a blank page for notes on what was learned and the great progress you made.

AWARENESS TRAINING

To know thyself is the beginning of wisdom.

— Socrates

Let's start with the most important training of all. Let's not call it work, in fact, let's call it a fun adventure, instead.

People call it exercise.

I call it conditioning, lengthening, realigning, balancing, each combined with body-awareness training.

There are plenty of teachers in these arts. I'm not providing you with a detailed day-by-day training plan. Who can for someone else, someone they haven't even met, about whom they know little other than they appear to have an interest in training for the toughest endurance sport there is, Aging.

My goal is to guide you toward the critical aspects of such training, much of which you can do unaided. Some of which is included in my online videos, on the *FitOldDog YouTube channel (link available at prepareforaging.com)*. Many instructors in physical fitness are young, and they have no personal experience with Aging. They only know the theory, if that.

I'm not a professional trainer, I've just been there, and learned a bunch of tricks that I'm sharing with you. I'm adding my five cents of experience, as I continue Ironman training with serious vascular disease in my mid-70s, along with my desire to avoid falling into the welcoming arms of Entropy, one second before I'm forced to do so.

This isn't easy, *you can't be chicken when you take this on (link available at prepareforaging.com),* it's a battle, and you want to be a warrior against Entropy, or you wouldn't be reading this book.

Fight well and long, my friend.

Much of what I know I learned over many years, and much of this will not apply to you. However, there are some critical keys to the process. Some common aspects for all doing battle with Entropy, as they face the ultimate endurance sport, Aging.

You have to learn slowly, wisely, intelligently, with appropriate education, especially anatomy. You will need at least a rudimentary understanding of biomechanics, or how we move our bodies. This can be gained from watching people, especially great athletes, children, who are already great athletes, and older people. Compare and contrast. Learn from the differences.

I might recommend more specific training, such as Feldenkrais, Pilates, Yoga, Gyrotonic, Continuum, weight training, even martial arts, each of which I've studied for a number of years, respectively. But if you are serious about your training, you will seek out the means to master the necessary skills, according to your age, budget, challenges and interests.

The objective of this book is not to provide you with a detailed workout plan to tell you exactly what to do. I'm just a guide, an experienced guide, pointing out the path you have to take. But it's you who has to walk your personal Aging journey, your personal battle with Entropy. It is your task to develop the best training plan for you. My task is to guide you on your journey toward becoming a multifaceted, anti-Entropy warrior.

- A flexible warrior.
- A realigned warrior.
- A balanced warrior.
- A conditioned warrior.
- A body-aware warrior.
- A socially and emotionally aware warrior.
- A warrior with a mission you love.

By taking this on, you become the hero in your own, personal hero's journey.

Imagine you are learning to paint, having never painted before. What do you do? You mess around with some paper and some paint. You don't try to become Matisse overnight.

You play. In fact, this is a great way to fight your nemesis, Entropy, who hates creative activities that cause you to live longer, better and happier.

Do the same with your body. Play around. See what you can find out about yourself, discover how your body works.

Think: What damage may I have done to myself to create tightness, weakness, imbalance, guarding, an important topic I'll address later? When you spot an issue, say to yourself, "Can I fix it?" "Do I need professional help?"

Here is the perfect example for you to consider, in *a short realignment video (link available at prepareforaging.com)*. I made that crude little movie eight years ago, with a Blackberry. Remember those? By the way, blackberries with soy creamer are really tasty.

I describe briefly below what is demonstrated in the video.

I noticed in the gym that I was sitting with my right foot resting on my left knee. I wondered, "What would it feel like to sit the other way around, with my left foot on my right knee?" It was almost impossible. I had to take my left foot in my hands and drag it up onto my right knee. It sure didn't want to go there. By sitting the same way around for 50-60 years, I had stretched my right hip muscles, ligaments, tendons and joints, and allowed those on the left to shorten and thus tighten.

This was a classic self-induced misalignment, destined to cause problems in my old age, if not corrected.

I fixed it over the next few years, by sitting both ways around. At first this was uncomfortable, to say the least. Now it is nearly balanced, after several years of work to repair multiple decades of lack of body-awareness.

How did I come to notice this issue in the gym, all those years ago? A single Feldenkrais lesson, described in the chapter entitled *Guarding*, woke me up to the importance of body-awareness training.

Your first goal is to become more body-aware, simply by watching how you and others move during daily activities.

Assess your body-awareness by *wiggling your finger and listening to your body's responses (link available at preparefor-aging.com).*

Not only will you gain information about yourself, you will gain essential knowledge, which leads to the wisdom needed to make progress, while reducing risk of injuries.

One last suggestion. I learned so much from years of Feldenkrais training, a significant amount of which I gained from a book, *Running With The Whole Body*, by Jack Heggie. Thirty daily exercises that will change your relationship with your body for ever. I suspect that the years of training contributed to my understanding of this excellent book, which is not just for runners. It's for anyone who wants to improve the way they move.

Highly recommended reading, when it comes to fighting Entropy.

That's your Aging training started. Well done! Starting is the hardest part. You looked in the mirror, you observed, you learned, you studied, you faced yourself as you are.

FLEXIBILITY TRAINING

The hard and stiff will be broken.
The soft and supple will prevail.

– Lao-tzu

It doesn't matter whether you were or are a star athlete, Aging is a sport you have yet to conquer. Look around at "old people." What is the first thing you see in 95+% of them?

Stiffness!

If you haven't worked out or stretched in ages, please avoid making the following common mistake.

———

I don't know how many people, mainly men, but not all, have told me how they'd realized they were getting out of shape and decided to return to the sport they loved in high school or college, be it running, basket ball, racquetball, or even pickle ball.

So they went to the track with their teenage son or daughter for a run, joined a pickup game of basketball with their homies, their term, not mine. Is it pejorative, I wonder? I've no idea. Or they went to the Y with a friend, who could knock their squash socks off, and within a week, a day or even a few minutes, they'd sprained an ankle, hurt their knee, or otherwise inflicted serious injury on themselves, to return forthwith, feeling sorry for themselves, feeling old, to tumble back into the welcoming, loving, open arms of Entropy.

———

They didn't follow the rules, and most likely strained a tight muscle, or a weak set of muscles caused their ankle to collapse on an abrupt turn.

Best to do some body-awareness work, including gentle exercise or safer still a massage from a sports masseuse to find areas of weakness, or have a physical assessment by a good physical therapist. Even though I was fit enough for a half-Ironman, of which I'd completed several, I had a full medical checkup before tackling the grueling physical challenges of a full Ironman race. I even had a sports physician run a cardiac stress test to be sure I could handle the training.

Do whatever preparation you can afford. Then fix any issues detected using gentle exercise, such as walking, followed by stretching. Stretching is better known as lengthening. Never stretch cold muscles, and consider all the other stuff I'm blah blah blahing about in this book.

I've only included things I consider essential.

STRETCHING

Let's briefly consider so-called stretching for building whole-body flexibility. You can find hundreds of stretching videos online, *one of which I made a while ago (link available at prepareforaging.com)*. But it's your body, your areas of tightness, your areas of weakness, so start with you. Just one tight muscle can screw you up, and your body contains hundreds of muscles for you to screw up. So be careful and don't over-stretch.

How to find areas of tightness on your own?

Look at yourself in the mirror, and watch how you move. Then sit or stand or walk or run, and look inside for tightness, look inside with your mind, your inner eye, your proprioceptive receptor machinery, whatever you want to call it.

Stop and listen to your body, it's talking to you. Poke around gently with your thumb to find tender muscles, because tight muscle are often sore and sensitive. Use pain as a tool to find tightness. Pain is generally your friend. If in doubt about this, ask someone with leprosy what they think.

Consider taking notes. My blog contains my notes. You could also blog your notes to help other people struggling against the ravages of that horror story known as Entropy.

Gently sway around, while looking in a mirror. Where do you find tightness or weakness. Some key areas to stretch are your shoulders, hips, especially hip rotators and hip flexors, quads and hamstrings. Take note of any tightness in your *psoas* muscles, as they can cause severe lower back pain, the cause of which is frequently misdiagnosed. A lot depends on your personal areas of tightness. Seek out assistance as need be, from a physical therapist or sports massage therapist.

Look down at your feet. Are they pointing straight ahead, or are they turned out like the feet of a clown. If it's the latter, you need to work on your tight lateral hip rotators, using the pigeon pose, carefully.

When it comes to tight muscles, a wonderful massage therapist told me years ago:

Underneath tightness lies weakness.

This is why "stretching" needs to be combined with effective conditioning or strength training.

By the way, how is your posture?

Are you standing erect, looking Entropy right in the eye?

Mr. Myagi, in The Karate Kid," was right. "Look in eye. Always look in eye." You don't think Entropy has eyes? You don't think Entropy is watching you, waiting for you to concede defeat?

Think again!

You've started stretching training and it's quite a trip that will free up your movements, to make you a more swift fighter against Entropy.

POSTURE TRAINING

Posture is an important tool for inviting more Syntropy into your life. I'm no expert and my posture sucked for years, but I'm much straighter and more upright now, after the painful, in fact agonizing, ministrations of my body-movement teacher, Rebecca Amis Lawson. I don't know how to describe what she did, and I think the only way for you to understand it is to go to a dance teacher, such as Rebecca, or at least watch this YouTube video Rebecca and I made a while ago, entitled, *FitOldDog Learning to Improve His Posture (link available at preparefor-aging.com)*.

NOTE: If you are comfortable in airplane seats, you have terrible posture.

Entropy loves airplane seats.

BALANCE TRAINING

Balance well to walk well, run well, swim well, and generally get around well. Let your body decay due to lack of exercise, as shown in the photo *on the website linked here (link available at prepareforaging.com)*lose your balance, fall down and break your pelvis, and you'll tumble nicely into the open arms of Entropy.

I practice balance daily, and I don't let blinding light impair my balance work, as is explained in the short story, below.

VISION MAKES US BLIND

I awake to a nice warm cat on my feet, a large warm dog huddled up to my side, and a wood stove needing attention. What's new?

Willbe, Cat and I would freeze pretty quickly in our tiny house without this little wood stove.

I go outside, one step away, to a world that is quiet and dark, with Orion's belt overhead. I step back into the growing warmth of our cosy little house, stand at the window, and do my routine balance exercise.

Standing, feet together, eyes closed.

Listening! I hear them all.

Those amazing balance sensors: somatic, inner ear, soles of my feet.

- **Somatic** *– Pressure on muscles, tendons, ligaments and joints, as my body sways around that straight line of gravity extending from outer space, through my body, to the center of the Earth. I guess it's not really straight, but I'll have to think about that in terms of all that Einstein relativity stuff. Let's assume it is straight, because it feels straight as a plumb line.*

- **Inner ear** *– The magic machinery of those semicircular canals, that tell me I'm upright and moving around gently, as my feet and ankles correct my center of gravity, with barely detectable muscle contractions and relaxations.*

- **Soles of my feet** *– Thousands of mechanoreceptors detect local pressure, vibration and shear, to tell my brain, maybe not even my brain, perhaps only local nerve pathways that pass through my spinal cord, to fine tune my position in space. Sensors to nerves to cord to nerves to muscles, adjusting their local tension.*

Then I open my eyes to see the stars, and I'm suddenly blind, elsewhere. My other senses of balance are overwhelmed by my powerful sense of vision. My mind automatically selects a light across the way, and locks in like a laser-guided missile. I immediately sway less, my stance is more solid, less fluid, less of a physical dance. My body becomes more rigid.

Our powerful sense of vision blinds us to the myriad of other balance systems in our bodies. Listening to all four of our balance systems is essential for effective balance training as we age.

───────

You might be stumbling around in the dark one day and take a fall because you neglected to train those non-vision-related, Syntropy weapons, your somatic sense, inner ears, and the soles of your feet.

There's value in going barefoot from time to time, as there is to mucking around in the garden soil with bare hands, as they both bring you back to the source, Mother Nature, the remarkable Biosphere, Gaia, the Syntropy-generating giant that nurtures us all.

So do your part for Mother Nature, train for Aging.

CORE TRAINING

Your hips, or pelvis, lie in a critical location, when it comes to body movement training and the necessary conditioning. Your hips join your upper body to your lower body, but they were really designed for a creature walking on all fours. I suspect this plays a role in all the problems they can cause.

Your hip bones, and their associated muscles, ligaments, tendons, nerves and other stuff, are bloody complicated. Sorry about that, but you need to know what you are dealing with. If you fail to respect your hips, you'll be in for lots of pain and other problems.

Core muscles: Pelvic floor, abdominal wall, back, and diaphragm muscles. And there are a bunch of them, including the all important medial and lateral hip rotators. Single leg calf raises provide a gentle core exercise, keeping your hips level, as you lift your body from the ball of one foot. The inactive foot is lifted from the ground by the work of your core.

Understanding your core is like understanding your car. You have two choices, as is so nicely explained in that important book, *Zen and the Art of Motorcycle Maintenance*, by Robert M. Pirsig. You can study and understand your body, to develop a quality relationship, or you can not do that, and trust your doctor. Best of luck with that, when it comes to body movement or muscular problems.

I won't attempt to write a discourse on the core machinery, I'll just say the following.

Entropy would love for you to give up trying to understand your core, to avoid the effort of learning a little anatomy, and working out how to make your core as strong as that of Rambo.

I guess you know what to do, now?

GUARDING TRAINING

It ain't what you don't know that gets you into trouble. It's what you know for sure that just ain't so.

— Mark Twain

THE SUMMER OF 2001.

In my late 50s, I was watching my youngest son, Nigel, compete in the Lake Placid Ironman. It was exciting, and I thought, "I'd like to do that." Little did I know what I was letting myself in for. A 2.4-mile swim, 112-mile bike ride, and a 26.2-mile marathon, all in one day. The biggest problem for me, was that I had never been a runner.

I didn't enjoy running in my youth. My legs lacked the stamina for it. Mild rickets as a toddler, due to vitamin deficiency, led to weak bones and joints. This was one of the effects of World War II. I was born in

1943, 18 months before the end of the war, with bombs dropping around the hospital at the time, I was told later. Even though Mum did a great job, food, especially good food, was scarce for the first 10 years of my life. War is hard on kids, and the nutritional injuries stay with you for a lifetime.

I had no idea how to engage my whole body in the process of running. I hired a coach and took lessons, increasing the distance. On reaching five miles, my right knee expressed extreme distress. Pain! The deep, throbbing, *"you-have-to-stop-running"* kind of pain.

Over the next year, I tried everything I could think of to cure that five-mile running-induced knee pain. Including the gold standard of rest, ice and stretching, plus pain relief gel and a heating pad. No luck!

This was followed by two chiropractors, a sports massage therapist, Yoga instructor, kinesiologist, acupuncturist, several podiatrists, including their expensive orthotics, two physical therapists, three sports physicians, a partridge in a pear tree, and the last physician diagnosed an inflamed bursa in my knee, into which he injected cortisone.

None of this made any difference. I still couldn't run more than five miles, pain-free. Furthermore, all this treatment cost a bundle. Over $3,000 dollars and nothing to show for it.

Then, I ran into Karen Dold. We knew each other from the world of science. Karen informed me that she'd abandoned molecular biology to teach the Feldenkrais Method. She explained that Moshe Feldenkrais suffered a serious knee injury while playing soccer. He studied his problem, and created a new method of movement therapy. Moshe used his approach successfully, to return to his beloved soccer.

The Feldenkrais Method is now used all over the world, to help people recover from injuries. Furthermore, both athletes and musicians use Feldenkrais to improve their performance.

"Can you fix my running-induced knee pain?" I asked. Karen replied that she would "give it a go." I arrived at Karen's house, expecting another failure for my $70.

Karen asked me to walk around her home office, while she watched. Then she said, "Stand in front of me, relax, and sway from side to side."

I did as instructed.

My understanding of the pains of body movement were about to change forever.

"Kevin, when you sway to the left your body remains straight? When you sway to the right, your shoulders rotate a little. Your right shoulder moves forward a few millimeters."

I looked down and there it was. But what did it mean?

Karen asked, "Have you had any serious accidents in the past?"

"I did have a motorcycle wreck about 40 years ago, which broke my right ankle."

"I suspect that you are guarding, or locking, that damaged right ankle. This forces your body to turn around your hips, as you sway to the right. Do you have more trouble balancing on your right leg?"

The jig was up.

I'd been guarding or locking that right ankle ever since my motorbike wreck. This impaired the movement efficiency of my right leg, making it hard to balance on that leg, throwing my body out of line. My knee pain was due to an issue with my ankle, believe it or not.

Unlike everyone else, including me, Karen didn't assume that pain in my knee meant the cause of my problem was in my knee.

Fixing my ankle fixed my knee pain. The pain in my knee was an action signal, and the action needed wasn't in my knee.

It was in my ankle, which is important for fine tuning one's sense of balance, while good balance is critical when running.

I worked to free up my right ankle, and before long I was running marathons, knee pain free.

Go Figure!

———

Beware guarding following any injury, including surgery, a strained muscle, tendon, ligament, bitten by a dog, even cheated in a relationship. Guarding is an overly extended protective reaction against such damage, and it needs to be turned off before it causes problems. Like my running-induced knee pain.

Entropy loves guarding, as it will slow you down, mess you up, make you want to give up whatever it was you were trying to achieve.

PHYSICAL TRAINING

Your body will respond to conditioning, training designed to strengthen your muscles, joints, bones, ligaments and cardiovascular system, heart and blood vessels. In the process, you condition your mind to fight that sly devil, Entropy.

The key to safe physical conditioning is to go slowly, listen to what your body has to say one and two days later.

Strength Training: Always warm up before doing strength training, for which I use an elliptical trainer. If you don't have an aortic aneurysm, I recommend a rowing machine. I sure miss it.

It will take a while for you to create your own strength training program. This can be done at home, but I prefer a gym because I learn from others, and it becomes a place where I train. It is best, as you age, to use weight training, rather than weight lifting.

I have workout routines I follow from memory, while you may need to ask an expert or find a routine you like online. I include, (a) strength training for my upper body, such as bicep curls, and bench or military press, You can look those up if you need to, (b) my core, mentioned previously, and, (c) legs, for which I include hamstring curls and squats, single leg calf raises, and a bunch of other stuff I've learned over the years.

You're serious about this? Yes? Go look this stuff up, or read a book on the subject. You can pose questions on my blog or one of my Facebook pages, if you want.

Make an effort, Entropy is watching.

Cardiovascular training: Here the goal is to get your heart rate up a bit, and that's basically it. Do this very slowly and carefully, and if necessary under medical guidance or supervision. My cardio training includes pushing effort in the pool, on the bike, or during the run. This is an art form that you need to take on.

Record your morning resting pulse each day, before getting out of bed. As I was Ironman fit in 2010, my resting pulse was 38 beats per minute, before I got that abdominal aortic aneurysm stent graft, which caused it to jump to 55, along with a severe increase in my previously normal blood pressure. These things happen when you have medical challenges, so adjust, ride it out, and get back on with life as best you can. You just have to work out how to get over it, as Entropy is waiting patiently beside you.

You're not dead yet, whatever Entropy would like you to think.

Make a controlled and steady effort, listen to your body, and get in shape. You could walk up a flight of stairs and note if you are out of breath. Then do some cardio training for a few weeks, and reassess the stair test. You'll see progress, that's for sure, if you do the work, and tell Entropy to buggar off.

Over-training: Watch for the signs, which include inability to sleep and an increase in your morning resting heart rate. If it's up more than five beats per minute, back off a bit.

I didn't learn this stuff over night, nor will you, but it's satisfying to see progress, and to know you are pissing off Entropy while delighting your friend Syntropy.

Do it!

And don't forget to stretch afterwards, for heaven's sake.

IMAGINATION TRAINING

Did you know it has been shown that if you imagine working out, conditioning muscles in your mind, that they actually do get stronger? This method is used for hospital patients following seriously invasive surgery to prepare them for movement once they are ready to escape from their hospital bed, and head for physical therapy, in order that they return to a normal life as soon as possible.

Don't underestimate the power of your imagination, when it comes to fighting Entropy.

NUTRITIONAL TRAINING

Remember, you are unique, just like everybody else.

– Margaret Mead

What you choose to eat is a valuable weapon in your fight against Entropy.

Fortunately, this is something you can do something about. But it is not as straightforward as the "so-called" experts would have you believe. No one can tell you the best foods for you, personally. There are some really bad foods, amongst which I include almost all industrial, highly processed products.

We are all different. Research studies generate average or statistical results. You are not a statistic, you are you. This is in the very nature of life. It's what allows any species to survive in response to major environmental changes. You are not identical to any other human being, which is why it is so important to listen to how your body responds to your food.

An optimal diet includes one you enjoy, which is a function of your upbringing, including your emotional history.

Educate yourself as best you can, and listen to your body, as it knows best.

Before you eat something ask yourself, "Would Entropy like me to eat this?"

HYDRATION TRAINING

WATER

Entropy is out to get you when it comes to hydration. If you don't drink enough water, especially when you age, you may suffer the ravages of vertigo, imbalance, risk of falling, even worse, fear of falling, stumbling into furniture, unable to stand as the room spins around, you can't reach the phone, you can't reach for water, you're alone with dehydration-induced vertigo, and the only way to fight off Entropy is with a calm mind, a slow progression toward the phone or your source of water, and if you fail you could well die.

How do I know that? I've been there, twice, once leading to a joy ride in an ambulance to the emergency room. Was it dehydration or a displaced rock in my inner ear? Who knows, who cares, I just dodged that dehydration bullet and the welcoming arms of Entropy.

Now I keep a supply of water and my phone close to my bed. Yep! I'm older.

Beware dehydration, my friend, because it's not your friend, it's the friend of Entropy.

BOOZE

This is a related drinking issue, as (a) alcohol is a diuretic, it makes you pee more, (b) it can make dehydration-induced vertigo and nausea much worse, and (c) if consumed to excess, excess being less and less the older you get, it gives Entropy superpowers by preventing you from training the next day or two. Alcohol is a muscle and brain poison, making exercise even more of a challenge.

Entropy loves that saying about "A hair of the dog."

I didn't instruct you not to drink alcohol or consume other drugs of choice. That's not my business. My business is encouraging you to fight Entropy with all your might. That doesn't mean you should never party.

My mantra is:

Everything in moderation, including moderation.

Hell, I've already ordered my annual English Christmas cake, which I'll consume with the odd glass of sherry, unless I have a hard workout the next day, in which case said cake and sherry will be consumed as a post-workout nutritional supplement.

As an anti-Entropy warrior, you'll know what to do.

EMOTIONAL TRAINING

The moment that judgement stops through acceptance of what it is, you are free of the mind. You have made room for love, for joy, for peace.

— Eckhart Tolle, *Practicing the Power of Now*

Entropy loves for us to carry around destructive "tapes" running in our heads. They drag us down, make life tougher than it needs to be, messes up our self-image, causes us to make not the best choices, and generally screw with our lives. I know, I've been there.

You need positive feelings to get you out of bed in the morning to do something. These are healthy emotions, or as Kahlil Gibran would say, they are the sails that drive your ship. He says, in the voice of *The Prophet*, that you also need a rudder to steer your ship, or your emotions will take you who knows where.

The key is to harness your emotions, while not letting them make your life hell, like my inappropriate sense of shame did for years. But I fixed it, and here's that story, which I also tell in a YouTube video, entitled, *Curing Inappropriate Shame Using Creative Visualization (link available at prepareforaging.com)*.

1953, BRISTOL, ENGLAND

When I was ten years old, I was pathologically shy and my family of origin, comprising Mom and five kids, moved house. Consequently, I had to attend a new school with class sizes of 50 or more, where I knew no one. In the middle of one unusually hot summer's day, after I had been at this school for a few months, my class, of roughly an even mixture of boys and girls, was lined up in the playground in rows for gym, with each of us standing about ten feet apart.

Unfortunately, I really needed to go to the bathroom, I needed to do number two. Now, there's a weird euphemism. I was too shy to ask to be excused, and then I did it anyway. There was my crap on the ground. I was wearing shorts, and boys of my age in England at that time hated to wear underpants.

Crap, literally!

The bizarre response to this event by the school staff was to call an ambulance and send me home wrapped in a blanket, while the whole school watched the excitement.

This experience was intensely traumatic for my young psyche, as you can imagine. From then on, if I thought about what had occurred in that playground, my heart would race, my face would redden, my hands would sweat, and I would feel really, really bad. I suffered severe feelings of shame and humiliation.

I'd built a destructive tape in my head, ready to run any time Entropy pressed the play button.

1993, CHAPEL HILL, NORTH CAROLINA, USA

I find myself, 40 years later, as a successful scientist, having raised a family, and still suffering intense private shame for that crappy event. It occurred when I was a 10-year-old kid. It made no logical sense. But it did make emotional sense. The experience was embedded in my psyche. It was part of who I was. I couldn't speak to anyone about this. It was too shameful. But then I encountered the concept of creative visualization, in a book of that name, by *Shakti Gwain*. I thought, "Great test case, let's give it a try."

I carefully followed the instructions in the book, setting the mental scene for my hoped-for cure. I imagined my 10-year old self, sweating it out in the playground. I imagined my older self, the me of 1993, placed back in England in 1953, near my old school. My older self, in my imagination, then walked up to the school just before the 'shameful event,' entered the hot playground, ignored by everyone, and located his distressed younger self.

My older self took my younger self by the hand to the bathroom, let him do his business in private, subsequently guiding him back to his spot in the playground. My older self then left the school the way he had come in, and the creative imaginary daydream ended.

It took all of two or three minutes, and to my surprise and amazement, I was cured of this inappropriate shame response. I still don't believe it, today. I'd cut that destructive tape, forever. I could talk about it, think about it, imagine it, and no shame response at all.

This is the remarkable power of the mind.

From then on, I was able to see this event in perspective. The emotional shame nightmare of 40 years was over. And now I am talking about it in this book, because I want to let you know that you do not have to let your childhood pain run your life.

You do have to access your inner child, and do some inner child work, if you want to fix such issues. I consider my inner child to be one of my best friends. In fact, I often feel like a 5-year old trapped in an old man's body.

Your inner child might be your best ally against the ravages of Entropy.

When it comes to fighting Entropy, your inner child can kick ass.

MEDICAL TRAINING

It's not safe to just blindly trust your doctor. Take their advice into consideration, of course, but you decide whether to put the pills in your mouth or not. Most of my experiences with doctors have been excellent, but here is an example of a doctor who helped me with a diagnosis, but I didn't take his pills. Nor should I have.

VALIUM? NO THANK YOU, DOCTOR.

About 15 years ago, I had severe pain in my ear. Thinking it was swimmer's ear, as I swim a lot, I went to a doctor for some antibiotics. The nice young physician looked in my ear and said, "It's not in your ear, Kevin; it's TMJ, jaw joint pain. Are you stressed about something? Grinding your teeth at night?"

As he spoke, the doctor started writing on his prescription pad. I agreed that my life had been difficult lately. I'd had trouble sleeping. I asked the doctor what he was writing.

It's a prescription for Valium, to calm you down, and a strong anti-inflammatory to protect that joint.

In response, I said, "I appreciate it, doctor, but no thanks. I'll take a week's vacation, meditate more, sleep a little more, and try to chill out. This is a warning sign that my life is out of control. A heart attack will be next, if I continue down that road." He insisted on handing me the prescriptions, which I later tore up and threw away. Within two weeks, following a drug-free treatment plan, my pain was gone.

It is important to be body-mind-aware enough to recognize valuable warning signs. Sometimes, you actually know better than your doctor.

Sure! Drugs can help us to continue a stressful lifestyle. And later take us toward something worse. Having veterinary training, I was aware of the addictive properties of Valium.

This knowledge contributed to a wiser choice, and I'm sure Entropy was not too pleased.

SPIRITUAL TRAINING

The unity of our Self is strengthened when we have a mission, when we are converging towards an attractor. When, on the contrary, we have no attractor cohesion diminishes, the chatter of the mind increases and our personality shatters.

— Ulisse Di Corpo, Antonella Vannini
An Introduction to Syntropy

I'm not the person who thinks about spirituality a great deal, so I won't talk about it much here, either. I'm sure you know more about your spiritual journey than I.

Do you mean wonder?

I've got plenty of that. The Universe is a remarkably exciting playground for the mind, so I play at understanding whatever I can.

When it comes to such things, no-one has the right to challenge your approach, as long as you do no harm to others.

Entropy will be only too happy to shatter your "faith" in your spiritual journey, so elect something that provides you with strong support.

That said, finding your mission in life can change everything for the better, as my work to help those with vascular disease and the challenges of Aging has for me.

COACHING

Sometimes you need a coach. When I attempted to qualify for the Boston Marathon, back in 2008, I sure needed my coach, Chris. I told him that I wanted to qualify for Boston, so he pushed me through a tough training schedule for about three months. It included 11 runs a week, with one long run.

Just before the race, Chris told me what he wanted me to do. He described a detailed race strategy based on my heart rate. It was magical. A plan I could never have devised. It worked, and I managed to qualify for the prestigious Boston Marathon.

I never could have done it without Chris, and some Syntropy of course.

There was something really valuable that came out of qualifying for Boston. It gave me confidence as a runner. Sometimes, during a tough training run or during an Ironman race, Entropy would say to me, *You're no runner,*

Kevin. Take a break. I could hear that destructive voice in my head.

I'd reply, "What the hell, I ran the Boston Marathon, of course I'm a runner."

And I'd run, both for myself and to piss off Entropy.

CONCLUSION: Sometimes you need a coach.

TAPERING TRAINING

For Ironman, the act of tapering is the gradual reduction of training intensity for several weeks before the race, so that on race day you are as strong as possible. At the end of an Ironman taper, I always feel fat and lazy, even though I never actually stop working out. I just do a lot less for a few weeks. That said, it's a tricky process that takes experience. Done right, you arrive at the start line, in that cold lake or the sea, fit as a fiddle, with no injuries and raring to go.

Any endurance sport, including Aging, benefits from tapering before an event. The only problem with the sport of Aging, is that you may not have a whole of lot time to taper properly.

YOUR EVENT MIGHT BE MAJOR SURGERY.

You've been learning all about your body through aware-ness training, and now you have to submit to anesthesia. This will fill you full of toxic chemicals, and then you'll be wounded by the surgeon's knife.

How do you taper for that? Well, you can't if it's an emergency surgery, but generally that is not the case.

When tapering for a planned surgery, go easy on yourself for a week or so, eat healthy and get plenty of sleep. Remove any noxious chemicals, such as alcohol, from your body, by drinking plenty of water. *The solution to pollution is dilution.* Work to put your body in tip top condition. Imagine you have a marathon to run, as major surgery is a marathon of anxiety, waiting, pain, and not being in control.

Done tapering?

Now comes the transition process.

TRANSITION TRAINING

Moving from one state to another is known as transition. In the Ironman, you transition from the comfort of your tent or hotel room, to sit in a cold lake before seven in the morning, when the gun goes off. This is followed by your transition from the swim to the bike, in a tent, a place of organized chaos, often six inches deep in mud, as you put your heavy wetsuit in a bag, and don your bike gear.

Try putting on wet socks under such circumstances. The bike to run transition is easier, but you forget something at your peril. For instance, fail to apply your sunscreen and you'll burn in the blazing sun. We train for this, over and over, until it becomes routine. It starts before the race, as you prepare your race bags, containing gear needed on race day. The final step is racking your bike, and then the die is cast. All that's left is a good nights sleep, carbs and plenty of water at 4:00

a.m., followed a power gel 15 minutes before the swim start.

When it comes to Aging, you will also face challenging transitions. Just getting out of bed with stiff muscles and joints is one. Being completely unable to read small print, or facing major surgery, are both transitions. For the former, you put your glasses in your Aging race bag, along with exercise, stretching, balance training, education, and all that other stuff, including a strong network of friends. We've covered that already.

HOW DO YOU TRAIN FOR THE TRANSITION TO SURGERY?

- By learning everything you can about the upcoming procedure.
- By meditating and otherwise calming your mind.
- By backing off a little on exercise, so your body is fully rested on surgery day (tapered).
- By following pre-surgical instructions to the letter, while understanding why they are important.
- By asking questions of your surgery team, so you are truly part of the team.
- By trusting your surgery team once the process begins. Your mood will effect the mood of the rest of your team, so provide them with a little Syntropy of your own.

Just like getting ready for an Ironman, really. Then you jump in the cold water, or onto the gurney.

HOW DO YOU TRAIN FOR THE OTHER TRANSITIONAL CHALLENGES OF AGING?

You get used to change by embracing change throughout life. What better time to start than now, if you haven't started already. Invite change into your life, by moving from one hobby to another. For instance, I have taken many courses at local universities for fun. One was in the Master's French program, another in mathematical modeling of biological systems. One I really enjoyed, which surprised me, was a drawing class, and then I've taken several classes on the art of writing. Taking on different sports also helped, as did changing jobs.

One change I hope you don't have to embrace, as it is painful, is divorce. Raising kids is another challenging but delightful change that taught me a lot. There are many ways to break out of old habits, and take the leap into a whole new life. For instance, do you enjoy your work? If not, I invite you to engineer a change for the better if you can.

Do such things, and when Entropy throws you another ringer, you will have no problem adapting, as you reach for a dose of Syntropy, to roll with the punches and take it in your stride.

You walk the walk. Anyone can talk.

RECOVERY TRAINING

The Ironman race is over, and it is time to eat and eat some more, let your muscles recover for a day or so, and plan your next race. It's that easy. For surgery, as you come around, there is this weird feeling of, "Where am I?" Then you remember. You don't feel any pain yet, but you will. It's normal. It's good pain. Pain to protect your surgery site and any internal damage. Time to recover, before moving, especially if you had an epidural. I forgot that one time, and ended up splayed on the floor.

Listen to your body, accept aid as needed, pain killers only if ABSOLUTELY needed, and recover. Then you can start thinking about exercise, as thinking about it actually does tone your muscles. Then start to think about the future, but first?

Be grateful!

Thank everyone who got you here, recovering.

You made it. Welcome back to the rest of your life, BUT:

You will have to learn how to live with whatever was done to you, as we people with aortic disease or PAD have to, so do it and get your life back on track.

Call up all the Syntropy you can, because Entropy will be waiting in the wings with a dose of post-surgical depression.

Piss off, Entropy, you say, *I've been trained for Aging.*

REWARDING

People like to say that exercise is its own reward. Buggar that! I like to reward myself after a race well run, progress made, Entropy slapped down, and so I do. Sometimes it's a bottle of beer handed to me by a friend after finishing an Ironman - don't tell me I didn't earn it, I finished a 140.6-mile race. Sometimes a dinner with friends, sometimes English Christmas cake and a glass of sherry, as I said before, to celebrate surviving the ravages of Entropy for another trip around the sun. Or does the sun go around us, I wonder? This an interesting philosophy Eigen vector squirrel question I think about from time to time. Don't you think about weird stuff, sometimes, too?

Reward yourself, and wake up the following day to plan your next race, effort, goal, kick Entropy's butt event.

TECHNOLOGY TRAINING

I'm forced to suggest that you consider some training in modern technologies. I work on a MacBook Pro, read on an iPhone, build websites and ebooks, use texting and email, and run a blog, a podcast that I don't really enjoy doing, several Facebook pages designed to help people with vascular disease, and I employ multiple online resources to advertise my books, including MailChimp, SurveyMonkey, BookFunnel, Twitter, Instagram and a range of search engine optimization tools along with anti-virus software.

I've mastered multiple tools for my work, including Photoshop and Pages for images, Vellum for book creation, and Adobe for video construction. I use online banking and purchasing systems, and infrequently make movie downloads. I do not walk around with a loud speaker blaring music and podcasts into my ear, which I consider to be unhealthy. I fight hackers daily, which is successful most of the time.

Can I do this all on my own? No! I seek assistance when I need it. For instance, I used an online for hire bidding service, Elance, and found a really great IT guy in India, Rojish. He's bailed me out a number of times, for a very reasonable price. I also employ companies to protect my websites from hackers, spammers and scammers.

You can't know everything, so track down the resources you need - before you get hacked.

How did I manage to learn all this stuff? One thing at a time. I took online courses, made mistakes, learned from my mistakes, accepted compliments and criticism. So I'm not being left behind by the technological revolution, and this allows my active participation in life as it is today.

Be left behind and Entropy will love you for it.

SOCIAL TRAINING

It is only too easy to become isolated as you age. You leave your workplace. Friends start to die off. I've lost several of mine. Younger people act as if you are in their way. Sometimes you are in their way, so don't do that. The answer is to be involved in a goal that is important to you, your life's meaning. This will bring you into contact with others.

It's also important to have friends of all ages.

I've managed to do that, even though I'm quite happy to spend a great deal of time alone, where I feel quite comfortable. I have friends and step kids, so their friends and family are in my life, including people ranging from teenagers to those in their 80s.

Entropy would love for you to become isolated.

LIVE YOUR TRAINING

I learned to live my training while studying the martial art form of Bruce Lee, Jeet Kune Do, in my late 40s. It was a blast. Bruce Lee was a remarkable athlete, so take a leaf out of his book:

EVERYDAY OPPORTUNITIES FOR EXERCISE

- *Take a walk whenever you can - like parking the car a few blocks away from your destination.*
- *Avoid taking the elevator; climb the stairs instead.*
- *Cultivate your quiet awareness by imaging your opponent* [Entropy] *attacking you - while you are sitting, standing, or lying down, etc. - and counter the attack with various moves. Simple moves are the best.*
- *Practice your balance by standing on one foot to put*

your clothes or shoes on - or simply stand on one foot whenever you choose [I forgot that I learned this from Bruce Lee].

— Bruce Lee, *The Tao of Jeet Kune Do*

Live your training but don't be obsessive about it, or you'll burn out.

Entropy loves burn out.

INTRODUCTORY TRAINING PLAN

In the end, it's your job to find the best way for you to undertake your Aging Training, and mobilize Syntropy to help you in your battle with Entropy. How you approach this training will depend on your age, health, finances and previous level of conditioning, physically, mentally, emotionally and spiritually.

Here's what I suggest as an initial three times per week, 30 minute, training plan, plus as much walking as you can manage. This is a minimal workout. Do this for several weeks, then make a more detailed plan based on where your issues lie, and what the hell it is you want to do with your life from now on.

As you increase your workouts, remember the 10% rule: never increase load, including intensity, effort, or distance, by more than 10% per week. If you are new to this, and really out of shape, you might consider a 5% rule.

1. **Awareness**: Look in the mirror, turn around and what do you see that might benefit from a little work, be it posture, belly fat, your self-image. Have a friend make a brief video of you walking, preferably when you are unaware. These short clips can be very revealing. You could also *wiggle your finger and see what happens (link available at prepareforaging.com)* (2 minutes).

2. **Flexibility**: Sit on the floor, reach toward your toes with one hand and then the other, keeping your back straight and chest out. Be gentle. I said toward your toes, don't force it, it's not necessary to reach them. Only go to where it is just a little uncomfortable. Stop there and turn your head from side to side. Feel what's going on in your body, especially hamstrings and hips. Watch for tight spots as you turn your head (2 minutes).

3. **Posture**: Have a friend make a video of you walking, watch said video every training day for this initial training period, and ask yourself, each time, "How's my posture, and how could it be better?" This will improve your posture and your powers of observation (5 minutes).

4. **Balance**: When standing in line, or at home if you prefer, unweight one foot, focus on balancing from your ankles. You can close

your eyes, too, if your balance is solid (2 minutes).

5. **Core**: Lay on your back, keep your lower back pressed to the floor and keep it there using pressure from your hands pushing into the floor on either side of your hips, bend your knees at right angles and sway them around, above your belly, tentatively extending your feet a little, while feeling the tension building in your lower abdomen or pelvis. This is exploratory, do not risk your lower back, and *if need be, watch my video (link available at prepareforaging.com)*. Look for tight spots in your pelvic area (2 minutes).

6. **Guarding**: Think back to an injury or surgery you've experienced. Imagine the pain you went through, and try to remember how you attempted to reduce this pain by tensing your chest or a particular part of an arm or leg, or tending to lean forwards or backwards. Workout what you did physically to ease that pain, and check to see if you are still doing it, even a little. If so, you've spotted a guarding reaction (3 minutes).

7. **Physical Training**: Do a wall squat, which means, lean your back against a wall, slide your back down the wall as you move your feet away from the wall, until you are in a sitting position, knees bent 90 degrees or less, depending on how safe you feel, where your

legs don't feel that they'll collapse. You are now being held up by the wall at your back and your powerful thigh and butt muscles. Stay like that for a minute, or until you can't stop the burn, and get back up without straining your lower back in the process (2 minutes).

8. **Nutritional Training**: Jot down what you ate each training day. That's it! Just jot it down. Now you know what you are eating. Make a note of why you ate what you ate, such as I like such and such, or someone told me it was healthy, or that's what my Mom used to cook, whatever. This is the first step toward nutritional awareness (3 minutes).

9. **Hydration Training**: Jot down each day a rough estimate of how much fluid you drank, including water, beer, sugary soft-drinks (not a good idea), whisky (subtract 40%). Make a note of why you drank whatever it was each time. This is the first step toward hydration awareness (3 minutes).

10. **Mental Training**: Do something that is mentally challenging that you have never tried before, be it a math problem, reading an article on philosophy, or learning three words in another language. This will keep your brain alive. It has to be something new to you, not something difficult that you are familiar with, that's the trick (3 minutes).

11. **Spiritual Training**: You are on your own with this one, as I'm no expert in spirituality or religion, but they seem to be really important to many people. I use daily meditation, vegetable gardening, and study through reading books, plus writing, to center my "soul." And I have a clear mission in life. Do something that seems important to you. I recommend quieting the mind meditation, for starters (3 minutes).

12. **Coaching**: Again, this is your call, as it will depend on your goals, issues, and finances. I've had some great coaches in both triathlons and body-movement training. This is up to you.

13. **Rewarding**: Choose your own reward, even if it's a beer or some sugary cake. It's your reward, not mine. I generally reward myself with a book.

Oh Yes! Don't forget to take the stairs, rather than the elevator, whenever you can, and stretch after every workout, whatever you do.

Entropy will hate that.

THE REST IS UP TO YOU!

Now choose a goal, create a training plan, make sure it's balanced across all areas, physical, mental, emotional, and spiritual.

Then tell Entropy to piss off, and say thanks to Syntropy or your life force, or negative Entropy, or God, or your guardian angel, or your mother, or whoever works for you.

NOW, DO IT!

May Syntropy be with you.

PAD PROGRESS REPORT

I started working on the final draft of this book several months ago. At that time, as described in the section, "MY DAY," I was struggling to overcome running and even walking-induced calf pain, due to the partially blocked popliteal artery in my right leg. Three months of fairly intense training, while working on the book, including 2x45min runs on a treadmill, several days per week, have provided considerable benefit.

I signed up for a local 8k (5-mile) run, in which I would have considered myself lucky to break an average pace of 16 min/mile.

Below are my mile times for that race:

Carrboro, NC, Gallop & Gorge, 8k run, 2019

Mile One - 15:07
Mile Two - 13:54

Mile Three - 13:56
Mile Four - 13:36
Mile Five - 12:56

Average pace per mile - 13:53

This is close to my target of 13:40 pace. Now to keep
training, so I can do that for 26.2 miles, to be ready for
the Florida Ironman in November, 2020. Yep! I
signed up.

There's no fool like an old fool!

Exercise is one of the most important health treatments
around, so please do it. I think that it might even be
more important than your diet.

Wishing you happy trails,

kev aka FitOldDog

ABOUT THE AUTHOR

Dr. Kevin Thomas Morgan is a retired veterinary pathologist, research scientist, avid Ironman-distance triathlete and aspiring writer. He works on ways to help older people keep going to enjoy every day they are lucky enough to have. He does this by writing books, creating instructional videos, and giving inspiring talks to groups of seniors. His current interests include reading and learning to write. He enjoys solving problems to help people in pain. Kevin is an enthusiastic vegetable gardener and vegan. Some of his work is designed to help people who, like himself, have aortic and other vascular diseases. He enjoys friends, family, his companion plants and animals, and not being dead for as long as possible.

RECOMMENDED READING

Chödrön P (2019). *Taking the Leap: Freeing Ourselves from Old Habits and Fears.*

Di Corpo, U, Vannini, A (2011). *An Introduction to Syntropy.*

Doidge, N (2007). *The Brain That Changes Itself: Stories of Personal Triumph from the Frontiers of Brain Science.*

Gibran, K (1923). *The Prophet.*

Gwain, S (1978). *Use the Power of Your Imagination to Create What You Want in Your Life.*

Hayflick, L (2007). *Entropy Explains Aging, Genetic Determinism Explains Longevity, and Undefined Terminology Explains Misunderstanding Both.* PLoS 3(12): e220

Hargrove, T (2014). *A Guide to Better Body Movement: The Science and Practice of Moving With More Skill And Less Pain.*

Harp, D, Feldman, N (1996). *Three Minute Meditator: 30 Simple Ways to Unwind Your Mind While Enhancing Your Emotional Intelligence.*

Heggie, J. (1996). *Running With the Whole Body: A 30-Day Program to Running Faster with Less Effort.*

Lee, B (1975). *The Tao of Jeet June Do.*

Pirsig, RM (2005). *Zen and the Art of Motorcycle Maintenance: An Inquiry Into Values.*

Tolle, E (2010). *The Power of Now: A Guide to Spiritual Enlightenment.*

✿ Created with Vellum

Printed in Great Britain
by Amazon